Liposuction

The Truth About Liposuction: An Introductory Guide to Surgery, Costs, Options, and What You Must Know

Table of Contents

Introduction

You've probably heard about "liposuction" at some point. Maybe you've heard about how it can completely change a person's appearance or about how it can add years a person's life. So, what exactly is "liposuction"?

This short and concise book provides introductory information regarding the topic of liposuction. The content here isn't meant to be a form of medical advice, as this book is meant for informational purposes only. In this book we are aiming to look at this topic in an unbiased light. We are not promoting liposuction, per se, but we want to make sure that if someone is interested in this controversial topic, he or she can reach more informed conclusions.

We will discuss the history of liposuction, the science behind it, other similar options, and how the operation can affect one's body. Most practically, we will look at the pros and cons of this medical treatment including what you can expect during and after treatment.

We hope that you are able to learn a thing or two from reading this!

Chapter 1:

What is Liposuction?

Liposuction, also known as lipo or lipoplasty, is the most common cosmetic procedure in the United Kingdom and United States. In fact, more than four hundred thousand procedures are done in the United States per year. It is a type of cosmetic surgery that involves breaking up and sucking fat from different parts of the body, usually in the thighs, abdomen, chin, neck, buttocks, upper and back of the arm, back, and calves. The fat is removed by using a hollow instrument called the cannula. The cannula is inserted under the skin, and a high-pressure vacuum is applied to the fat.

Liposuction is typically performed as an outpatient procedure in a hospital, doctor's office, or ambulatory surgery center. Generally, patients do not need to stay in the hospital overnight, unless they need to remove a huge amount of fat. In many cases, the procedure involves the use of local anesthesia, and patients may or may not be provided with a sedative. Deep sedation with local anesthesia or general anesthesia may be used when dealing with a large volume of fat.

It is important to note that liposuction is neither an obesity treatment nor a weight loss method. It does not get rid of cellulite, stretch marks, or dimples. It simply changes and enhances the contour of the body. Those who undergo the procedure generally have a stable weight but want to get rid of unwanted fat deposits in certain regions of their body.

Liposuction can permanently take away fat cells from the body, as well as alter its shape. However, it can also cause the remaining fat cells to grow bigger if a patient does not maintain a healthy lifestyle. Also, there is a limit to how much fat can be removed. If not done properly, then the procedure can result in infections, scarring, dents, and lumpiness in the skin. Nevertheless, liposuction can also be beneficial for certain medical conditions, such as lipomas, gynecomastia, and lipodystrophy syndrome.

In recent years, liposuction techniques have been improved to make the procedure less painful, safer, and easier for the patient. These new techniques are as follows:

Ultrasound-Assisted Liposuction

Ultrasound-assisted liposuction uses a special cannula that rapidly vibrates to give off ultrasound energy, which liquefies fat, making it much easier and faster to remove. It is useful in removing excess fat in the back, upper abdominal region, and sides. In general, two types of ultrasound cannulas are used: a solid probe, which creates a pool of tumescent solution and emulsified fat beneath the skin, and a hollow-core probe, which emulsifies and removes fat.

Tumescent Liposuction

Tumescent liposuction involves the usage of a local anesthetic to numb the part of the body in which the tube is supposed to be inserted. It also involves the injection of an anesthetic solution that contains lidocaine and epinephrine into the fatty tissues prior to the procedure. Using general anesthesia may no longer be necessary.

Laser-Assisted Liposuction

Laser-assisted liposuction involves the use of low-energy waves to liquefy fat. Once liquefied, the fat is removed with the use of a tiny cannula.

Super-Wet Liposuction

Super-wet liposuction is similar to tumescent liposuction, except that it uses less fluid, which is about the same amount as that of the fat tissue and the fluid removed. This procedure usually requires the use of IV-epidural or general anesthesia and takes one or two hours to perform.

Power Liposuction

Power liposuction involves the use of a motorized cannula, which is moved back and forth very rapidly over a distance of three to five millimeters. This method can remove forty percent more fat per minute as compared to manual liposuction. It is much faster to complete and has smoother results.

What to Keep In Mind Before The Procedure

Prior to your treatment, see to it that you eat properly. Proper nutrition and hydration are necessary to prevent you from bruising easily. Additionally, it is important to maintain the right kind of diet in order to avoid additional stress from the surgery. Remember that stress can weaken your immune system, slow down the healing process, and cause fatigue. Therefore, you need to make sure that your body receives adequate amounts of the following:

Vitamin C

Vitamin C improves your body's ability to heal. It is also an antioxidant, which is why it is effective in eliminating toxins, fighting against bacterial infections, and protecting your body against allergies. Vitamin C is also necessary for repairing collagen and reducing the incidence of blood clots.

Iron

Iron increases red blood cell production, prevents fatigue, and maintains your natural skin tone.

Zinc

Zinc speeds up the healing process of external and internal wounds, as well as promotes the repair and growth of tissues. It also increases mental alertness and fat metabolism.

B vitamins

These essential vitamins repair tissues, relieve pain, and maintain the nervous system. They also promote healthy blood vessels, skin and nails, reduce water retention and promote circulation.

Dos and Don'ts Before the Procedure

Dos:

Eat the right kinds of food.

Drink milk or eat dairy products.

Eat lean cuts of meat, such as lamb, beef, or poultry.

Have a medical examination. Go to your doctor to have a physical exam about two weeks before your surgery to ensure that you are in good health.

Don'ts:

Have a monotonous diet.

Consume alcohol during the twenty-four hours before your surgery.

Use recreational drugs.

Use anti-inflammatory medications or medications that contain aspirin one month before your surgery.

Take more than 200 mg of Vitamin E.

Take garlic pills. These pills can thin blood and cause excessive bruising.

What Can You Expect After The Treatment?

After going through the liposuction procedure, the affected area will be wrapped firmly to lessen the pain, swelling, and bruising. Depending on the part of your body that underwent the procedure, you will use an elastic bandage and tape, special girdle, support hose, or a firm-fitting garment.

Your surgeon may require you to wear the wrap or compression garment for at least three weeks. During the first week or two, you may notice some bruising, swelling, and some fluid in the incisions for a while. In order to prevent infections, you may use antibiotics.

If you are worried about missing work or school, do not worry, as you can get back to doing what you used to do as soon as your treatment is over and once the effects of sedation or anesthesia wear off. This may take several days or even weeks, though. If your treated area is quite large, then your recovery time may be longer. You may want to stay home and avoid moving around too much during this time to avoid complications.

Why Do People Undergo Liposuction?

People mainly undergo liposuction to reshape certain areas of their body, particularly those that did not respond to exercise and diet. In women, these areas often include their hips and their outer thighs. In men, such areas include their back and their waist. Other common areas that go through liposuction include the neck, face, abdomen, buttocks, legs, and upper arms.

In some cases, liposuction is performed along with other cosmetic surgical procedures like a face-lift, tummy tuck, or breast reduction. Liposuction is also useful in treating medical conditions, such as benign fatty tumors, issues with fat metabolism, abnormal enlargement of breasts in men, and excessive sweating of the underarm region.

How Well Does Liposuction Work?

The procedure is usually effective in removing fat deposits in different areas of the body. However, if you gain back the weight after a while, the areas where fat was removed will become fat again. In some cases, the fat appears in another area of the body.

Immediately after the procedure you will notice great improvements in your body's contour. Such improvement may continue for a few more weeks or months. The total effects of liposuction may only be seen after a few more months. In some cases, it takes a year for the full effects to show.

The skin at the treated area does not become tighter, except if you undergo laser liposuction. Once the fat is removed from a certain area, the skin surrounding it may become loose. It may take half a year before the skin becomes tighter around that area.

Also, you have to keep in mind that the human skin varies greatly. Some people have highly elastic skin that retracts quickly, while others have looser skin. Young people usually have more elastic skin than older people. This is one factor in why some women get tons of stretch marks during pregnancy while others do not, even if they gained the same amount of weight. Skin elasticity is a genetic factor.

What Are The Risks Involved In Liposuction?

If done correctly, liposuction is a generally safe procedure. However, if multiple areas require treatment, you may be at risk of more complications. Some of the possible side effects associated with liposuction are:

Permanent skin discoloration

Temporary pain, bruising, puffiness, and numbness in the treated area

Some blemishes, irritation, and scars around the sites of incision

Swelling or saggy skin

Rough skin surface

Nerve and skin damage

Growth of fat around organs, like the liver or heart

After undergoing liposuction, make sure to do your best to keep the weight off. If you re-gain the weight, then fat may re-appear on the areas where they had been removed or appear in different areas of your body. However, fat may also develop around your liver or heart, and this can be dangerous to your health.

Other Complications:

Aside from fat appearing around certain organs, you may also develop the following complications:

Blood or fat clots that may affect your lungs, which may be life threatening

Excessive fluid loss and blood loss, which can lead to shock

Fluid buildup inside the lungs

Infections

Toxic reaction to the solution used

Rupture in the cavity that holds the organs in the abdominal region

Organ damage

Note: Liposuction is not ideal for people with severe heart problems. It is also not advisable to those who are pregnant or are suffering from blood-clotting disorders, such as thrombophilia.

Chapter 2:

History of Liposuction

The first recorded use of liposuction was in the 1920's by Charles Dujarier, a French surgeon. He developed the concept of fat removal and body contouring. However, his interest in such concept was lost after conducting a failed procedure. Dujarier performed an operation that eventually caused gangrene in the patient.

In the 1970's, interest in liposuction was once again ignited when European surgeons made use of primitive curettage techniques. They tried to sculpt fat buildup with the use of a curette, which is a surgical tool for scraping. However, the results were inconsistent, causing such interest to be lost again. There were also been blood clots, unevenness of the skin, abscesses, and a variety of other health complications during this uncertain period. Some doctors even tried to reshape the body by surgically removing both the skin and fat. This caused unsightly scarring and the re-accumulation of fat around the sites of incision, which eventually resulted in physical deformity.

Eventually, in 1974, Arpad and Giorgio Fischer, father and son Italian gynecologists, developed the blunt tunneling technique that became the basis for modern liposuction. They used a blunt and hollow instrument known as the cannula. This surgical tool enabled them to create tunnels between the major blood vessels of the body as they sucked fat out.

By 1978, liposuction rose to popularity when French surgeons Pierre Fournier and Yves-Gerard Illouz started to focus on the work of the Fischers and made certain improvements to the equipment. Seeing the potential impact of the procedure, Illouz introduced it to the public and then developed the "wet technique," which involved injecting a solution of salt water into the fat before suctioning it in order to make the process easier and reduce bleeding.

The Illouz Method presented a suction-assisted method for getting rid of fat cells. The solution was injected into tissue using cannulas. The fat deposits were broken down and removed with the suction device. This technique showed low morbidity and high reproducibility.

Pierre Fournier also pioneered the use of lidocaine as a local anesthetic, which laid the groundwork for the tumescent technique used today. He also modified the surgical incision method and used compression techniques post-surgery. Instead of having just one or two incision sites, he used a crisscross method that involved several incision sites to give more contouring. According to him, the application of compression to the treated area could better support it, as well as shape the suctioned tissue.

In the 1980's, liposuction has started to become popular in the United States. However, a lot of patients experienced skin rippling and excessive bleeding after the procedure, so liposuction gained negative publicity. Some of the first American doctors to perform liposuction were Rhoda Narins, a dermatologist in New York, and Richard Dolsky and Julius Newman, plastic surgeons who directed a liposuction course.

In 1985, Dr. Jeffrey Klein, a dermatologist in California, revolutionized liposuction by using the tumescent technique, which involved the injection of epinephrine and lidocaine into the fat. It diminished the need for general anesthesia. Liposuction could be performed with just local anesthesia and a smaller cannula. Patients did not have to worry about undesirable skin conditions or excessive bleeding. This more refined method has quickly become the favored procedure for women when it comes to shaping their thighs and buttocks.

In 1992, Michele Zocchi, a professor in Italy, presented Ultrasonic-Assisted Lipoplasty (AUL) as an alternative to standard cannula suction. He wanted this technique to allow for the execution of liposuction without damaging the veins and nerves that were usually destroyed with the use of a blunt cannula. This procedure involved the use of ultrasonic energy, which was applied to the fat cells before suctioning. AUL was initially a hit in Europe and South America. However, it was eventually rejected when a number of patients complained of burns, peeling, and buildup of fluid in the treated area.

At the end of the 1990's, the use of ultrasound for liquefying fat was introduced. Such developments have resulted in liposuction technique improvements over the years. In 1997, the American Society of Plastic and Reconstructive Surgeons supported the ultrasonic liposuction and developed a series of courses to teach members on how to use this new technology properly. However, dermatologists rejected it because they thought that it had more complications than benefits.

In 1998, Power-Assisted Lipoplasty (PAL) was approved, even though it was considered to be significantly different than traditional liposuction. This method involved the use of a customized cannula that pulsed while it suctioned. Today, it is easy to remove fat without much pain, loss of blood, and other complications. The development of liposuction throughout its existence has definitely seen its share of peaks and valleys, leaving us with a much-refined process that minimizes side effects and optimizes   results.

Chapter 3:

The Science Behind Liposuction

As mentioned earlier, liposuction can improve the contours and shape of your body by suctioning undesired localized exercise and diet-resistant fat deposits. Even though it is not a substitute for exercise and dieting, it can still remove the stubborn areas of fat that do not respond to the traditional methods of weight loss.

Laser Liposuction

Many patients prefer this method because it does not possess the risks of surgical procedures, such as a tummy tuck. They also like the fact that it can be combined with standard liposuction. Laser liposuction is a minimally invasive treatment that melts fat with a laser. It offers the additional advantage of creating new collagen for the skin. The laser also causes collagen contraction, and thus, tightening the skin and preventing it from sagging.

Additionally, laser liposuction can remove more fat when compared to standard liposuction.

A lot of women who undergo standard liposuction usually notice their skin sagging when the fat is taken away. Dr. Abbas Chamsuddin, from the Center for Laser and Interventional Surgery, said that fiber-optic laser might be applied to different areas of the body. He added that it could excellently sculpt tight skin.

The procedure of liposuction has already been popular for over two decades. A lot of people, however, are still hesitant to try it due to their fear of having sagging skin. People who wish to get rid of their abdominal fat are especially discouraged because they need their skin to retract. That being said, standard liposuction has limits when it comes to volume.

Fortunately, a combination of standard liposuction and laser lipolysis can result in amazingly sculpted bodies without sagging skin. This procedure can help people get rid of their belly fat and still have tight skin afterwards. Laser liposuction is ideal for multiple parts of the body, such as the arms, neck, breast, thighs, calves, love handles, and belly. Patients must have their measurements taken and recorded prior to the treatment.

What About Lipoglaze?

Lipoglaze, or cryolipolysis, has been clinically proven to reduce fat cells permanently by freezing. It is actually a non-invasive and non-surgical alternative to liposuction. This method targets and reduces fat without damaging the surrounding tissue. It works well on stubborn areas of the body that do not respond to exercise and diet alone.

This makes it the most ideal solution for attaining the body you have always wanted without having to turn to expensive and painful treatments. When you go through lipoglaze, your fat cells will be eliminated forever.

The fat cells in your body begin to crystalize once they are exposed to precise cooling. This causes your body to reject such cells naturally and pass them out through your lymphatic system. You can eliminate up to thirty-three percent of fat with this procedure.

Lipoglaze is quick, painless, effective, and discreet. You do not have to worry about any downtime. You can actually undergo treatment during your lunch break. There is no need for you to take a rest day, so you can immediately get back to work after the procedure.

Within two to eight weeks, you will start to see results. The number of sessions you need to undergo depends on the density of your fat cells and the area that requires treatment.

Chapter 4:

The Effects of Liposuction

It cannot be stressed enough that to maintain the fat loss from liposuction, a person has to maintain a healthy diet and exercise on a regular basis. In context, liposuction is still generally considered a safe and effective procedure. It can also be easily combined with cosmetic surgery techniques, which can greatly improve a person's looks and self-confidence.

Positive Effects of Liposuction

Better Health

Removing fat from your body can have positive effects on your overall health. Many doctors agree that weight loss is an effective way to reduce the risk of heart disease, diabetes, and certain types of cancer. Even though liposuction cannot get rid of massive amounts of fat, it is still useful in eliminating stubborn fat pockets that may weigh up to ten pounds.

Liposuction is also beneficial for people who need to undergo breast reduction. This breast surgery method is useful when the patient's very large breasts put him or her at risk of health issues, such as headaches, back pain, and neck pain.

Better Appearance

The contouring and smoothing effects of liposuction can make one look and feel much better about their daily life - your clothes might fit you better and you might look more ideal in your mind. Many people have reported that they feel confident in public after previously feeling shy and hesitant to be seen.

Fat Removal

Each cell in your body has a particular function that is crucial for your overall health. Fat cells store unused energy from the food you consume. Your body uses fat for shock absorption, insulation, and fuel. However, excess fat cells may have to be removed to eliminate unwanted fat on certain areas of your body. Once a fat cell is created in the body, it stays there for good, and the good news here is that once fat cells are removed via liposuction, those cells are gone for good.

Cellulite Removal

Fat cells that push through the collagen cause cellulite, which tends to be more common in women than men. As an added benefit, liposuction can help remove cellulite. However, one should keep in mind that a permanent cure for cellulite does not exist. You cannot rely on liposuction to remove cellulite from your body, but it could possibly happen.

Negative Effects of Liposuction

Skin Numbness

You may lose sensitivity in the treated area for two to four months. In some cases, however, the numbness can be permanent.

Loose Skin

Your treated area may have loose skin after the procedure. Skin generally regains its firmness after about six months, but if your skin does not get firm on its own, then you may need surgery to get rid of the excess skin.

Fat Metabolism Syndrome

Although rare, fat metabolism syndrome can be serious. It can cause permanent disability or even death. It occurs when parts of the loosened fat tissue get stuck in a blood vessel. If not treated immediately, the fat then moves to the brain and lungs, causing brain damage and damage to the lungs and cardiovascular system. This is just one reason why it is important to go for post-op check-ins to monitor your full recovery.

Continual Low Self-Esteem

While low self-esteem is certainly not a direct effect of liposuction, it is important to note that a certain percentage of people view procedures like liposuction or plastic surgery as a "cure all" to the big problems in their lives. This is a dangerous road to go down because it usually is based on delusion. While liposuction can certainly improve your physical appearance, and in turn your self-image, it is essential that you also take active steps to build a life that provides you happiness in other ways than from the way you look.

This means adressing the deep-rooted issues rather than only the superficial issues of your self-image. Many people blame the procedure for their unhappiness in the way they look, failing to realize that they underwent it with unrealistic expectations.

Chapter 5:

Traditional Liposuction Compared to Smart Liposuction

Traditional liposuction involves the use of general anesthesia, which is administered through an IV and puts the patient to sleep. It is also typically performed in surgery centers or hospitals. In this procedure, large incisions are made in the areas that require treatment. Such incisions must be large enough to accommodate the cannulas. The cannula is moved under the skin with a jabbing motion to remove the fat from between the muscle and the skin.

The downtime of traditional liposuction depends on how much fat was removed. The patient may be required to stay in the hospital or be on bed rest. Swelling and bruising may also be noticed during recovery. The discomfort and pain can last for a few weeks, and patients are usually asked to wear a compression garment for up to six weeks.

Smart liposuction, on the other hand, is a revolutionary version of liposuction. It removes fat with the use of a laser. As it is less invasive than traditional liposuction, it has fewer side effects. During smart liposuction, the body of the patient excretes fatty oil through his or her liver. The United States Food and Drug Administration approved the use of SmartLipo, the first laser-assisted liposuction procedure, in 2006.

Laser-assisted liposuction works on localized and small areas of fat on the body and face. However, just like any other surgical procedure, it may not be ideal for everyone. You must be in good shape and have a normal body weight to qualify for the procedure. You must also have areas of fat that do not respond to diet and exercise alone.

Smart liposuction starts with a consultation where the doctor will ask about your medical history and evaluate the areas that you want to treat. Before undergoing the procedure, you will be given local anesthesia. Then, your doctor will make a one-millimeter incision in your skin and insert a cannula with a laser fiber under your skin. The cannula will be moved back and forth in a fanning motion.

Depending on how much fat was removed from your body, you may be advised to stay home and recuperate for one to two days. Afterwards, you can go back to work or school. You just have to avoid performing strenuous physical activities and taking a hot bath for a couple of weeks. It is also advisable for you to wear a compression garment for a week to speed up the healing process. You may be asked to wear close-fitting elastic garments to help reduce swelling.

Traditional Liposuction vs. Smart Liposuction

Traditional liposuction can treat large areas, but it cannot fix loose or sagging skin. However, smart liposuction works well on loose skin. Traditional liposuction is most ideal for treating the thighs, buttocks, abdomen, hips, and breasts of men. Smart liposuction can help treat the face, neck, jowls, arms, loose skin, and breasts of men.

Traditional liposuction requires local, general, or epidural anesthesia, while smart liposuction only needs local anesthesia. Traditional liposuction can cause bruising, bleeding, dimpling, infection, and rippling under the skin if too little or too much fat is removed. It may also cause blood clots, swelling, fluid accumulation, nerve damage, and even death. Smart liposuction can cause soreness and minor bruising.

After the procedure, traditional liposuction can result in pain, burning, or soreness for several days or weeks. The swelling may continue for up to six weeks, and the stitches may dissolve after ten days or so. While in recovery, one must avoid performing strenuous physical activities or exercises for a month. Smart liposuction can cause minor discomfort. You may go back to your regular activities within one to two days, but you have to avoid performing strenuous physical activities for two weeks.

Traditional liposuction can cost two thousand to seven thousand dollars per body part, and smart liposuction can cost four thousand to eight thousand dollars.

Why Choose Smart Liposuction Over Traditional Liposuction?

Smart liposuction offers better results with much less downtime. Moreover, it gives the additional benefit of tightening the skin, which other techniques cannot give. There are three laser wavelengths used during the smart liposuction procedure:

1440nm

This wavelength is attracted to the fat, so the laser melts it away.

1320nm

This wavelength is attracted to water in the skin tissue. It sends signals to your brain to produce new elastin and collagen, as well as to thicken and tighten the skin tissue. It also causes the skin to lighten.

1064nm

This is the final wavelength, and it cauterizes the blood vessels in order to protect the skin against blood loss and tissue trauma.

Smart liposuction has minimal downtime and pain. After the procedure, you will not feel any pain or major discomfort. You can actually drive yourself home and do chores. However, for the next few days, you can expect some soreness. Do not worry because such soreness is mild, as if you have just finished a rigorous workout regime. You may also have some bruising and swelling. However, this is minimal and typically goes away after a few weeks.

Chapter 6:

The Future of Liposuction

Liposuction is undoubtedly one of the most popular cosmetic surgery procedures, and ongoing research is always being conducted in order to make it even more effective and efficient. In fact, its predictability and safety took a huge leap forward with the introduction of wet techniques, such as tumescent liposuction. Due to such innovation, liposuction has become more acceptable in society.

In the future, it is expected for liposuction to have the capability to noticeably improve skin condition. Most patients' skins are elastic enough to have good post-surgical results. Those with looser skin may require other surgeries to have positive results in this area.

Likewise, it is expected that minimally invasive liposuction that involves the use of lasers to replace tummy tuck procedures in melting fat. Tummy tuck can be combined with standard liposuction to reap the benefits of laser lipolysis and produce new collagen. As you know, collagen is a protein that provides the skin its texture and tone.

In addition, the laser causes the collagen to contract and tighten the skin. Such tightening of the skin reduces the odds of sagging, which is a common side effect of standard liposuction. Also, laser lipolysis allows for the elimination of more fat compared to standard liposuction.

Dr. Abbas Chamsuddin, an interventional radiologist at the Center for Laser and Interventional Surgery in Georgia, said that most of the women who go through standard liposuction become discouraged when their skin sags after the removal of fat. Even though liposuction has been in existence for over twenty years, a lot of people are still reluctant to try it because they do not want their skin to sag after the procedure. Hopefully, the next decade will see a big improvement in this regard.

Also, traditional liposuction has limitations when it comes to how much fat can be removed. So, in order to prevent skin from sagging, fiber-optic lasers can be used during laser lipolysis. It sculpts the body and tightens the skin. Chamsuddin adds that combining laser lipolysis with standard liposuction can result in excellently sculpted bodies with tight skin.

The Advent of Nano Liposuction

Liposuction techniques continue to evolve, and one of the most recent concepts involves the application of nanotechnology toward body contouring. Professors at the University of California and the University of Nevada School of Medicine are developing nano liposuction, which makes use of gold nanoparticles.

When these gold nanoparticles are exposed to laser light, they start to melt the fat. Some of the supposed benefits of this procedure include less risk of collateral damage and less contour irregularities. Because the fat melts at a lower temperature than its surrounding tissues, there could be less collateral damage within the area. The fat cells are also melted instead of being broken apart, therefore reducing any concerns regarding contour irregularities.

Conclusion

Thank you for reading this! We hope this short, concise book was able to teach you a thing or two about the intriguing liposuction treatment.

Now that you understand the important factors regarding liposuction, you can decide if you want to try it, or if you can inform your friends who ask you about it. Plus, a little addition to your knowledge doesn't hurt, right? Our world is becoming increasingly interested in the use of this incredible tool, whether it be for substantial weight loss, improved health markers, or as medical assistance to those who need it.

If you've learned anything from this book, please take the time to share your thoughts by sending me a personal message, or even posting a review on Amazon. It would be greatly appreciated and I try my best to get back to every message!

Thank you and good luck in your journey!

www.ingramcontent.com/pod-product-compliance
Lightning Source LLC
Chambersburg PA
CBHW070941180526
45168CB00003B/1130